Rx 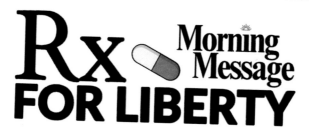 Morning Message
FOR LIBERTY

An Exclusive Signed Copy

Jeffrey I. Barke, M.D.

Introduction

We have been taught for a generation that the foods our grandparents ate are unhealthy. Instead, we are encouraged to consume highly processed and nutritionally vapid products. These new and improved choices have led to chronic illnesses, including obesity, diabetes, hypertension, cardiovascular disease, and even cancer. Our media is saturated with food companies and big pharma ads, and our healthcare industries are captured by their pharmaceutical sponsors.

I received only a few hours of nutrition education during my medical school training – mostly about obscure diseases such as scurvy, beriberi, and rickets. We were taught that red meat was unhealthy, butter clogged our arteries, and butter substitutes made with vegetable oils were healthier. We were told that low-fat diets should be emphasized to patients to prevent heart disease and diabetes. Yet, 150 years ago, heart disease and type 2 diabetes were much less common.

Heart disease is now the leading cause of death in the United States, and 40% of our population has a chronic disease. Just look around the next time you are at the mall – how many obese and unhealthy-appearing people do you see? Now, look at the old pictures of the Woodstock music festival from the summer of 1969; you can't find a single obese person in the pictures.

It was during the Covid crisis that I realized much of our modern allopathic medical focus has been wrong and perversely influenced by big pharma's need to feed their bottom line. A disease model that says there isn't a symptom or condition that a pharmaceutical product cannot help is a model that thrives on illness. We are one of only two countries that allow direct-to-consumer advertising by the pharmaceutical industry.

1

During the Covid pandemic, I started posting and recording on social media, particularly on Instagram, under the handle @RxForLiberty. I shared information on a radical new path: a return to a more foundational approach to health that emphasizes clean eating – grass-fed organic meat, including organ meat; raw dairy; raw honey; organic produce; pasture-raised eggs; sun exposure; hydration with purified water; exercise; and a focus on mental health and stress reduction.

To my delight, my presence on social media grew, and my reach expanded. During this time, my office-based medical practice was filled with patients seeking out a like-minded physician – one who respected a patient's right not to be vaccinated and never required a useless face covering. My Instagram "Morning Messages" became a go-to source for holistic health ideas for many people.

Thanks to the encouragement of my children, I have embarked on this journey to publish my insights in the form of a Morning Message book. My daughter, Allie Barke, created my Instagram account and my website. My son-in-law Pierce McDonnell and Sam Barke my son, offered to help me publish this book. I hope you enjoy this book as much as I enjoyed creating these messages. Thank you for inviting me on your journey toward optimal health of the mind, body, and soul.

Jeffrey I. Barke, M.D.

About
Dr. Jeffrey Barke

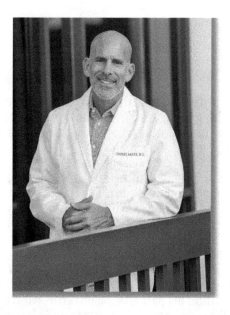

Dr. Jeffrey Barke has been a board certified primary care physician in private practice for over 25 years. He completed his medical school and family practice residency at the University of California, Irvine. He has served as an Associate Clinical Professor at U.C. Irvine and a Board Member of the Orange County Medical Association. Dr. Barke is a commissioned officer in the US Army Reserve Medical Corps. He is also a reserve deputy and a tactical physician for a local law enforcement SWAT team.

Dr. Barke also served as an elected School Board Member for the Los Alamitos Unified School District for 12 years and is the Co-Founder and current School Board Chair of a free public charter school in Orange, CA called Orange County Classical Academy that uses Hillsdale College's curriculum. Dr. Barke is the author of COVID-19, A Physician Take on the Exaggerated Fear of Corona Virus. He is a sought-after speaker on the failure of government education and all things related to COVID-19.

Dr. Barke is a proud founding member of America's Frontline Doctors.

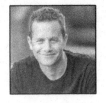

Forward Written by Kirk Cameron

With joy and gratitude, I wholeheartedly recommend this book as a personal health guide. Dr. Barke is not only a great doctor but also a friend and a guiding light toward holistic wellness, deeply valuing the importance of nurturing your body, mind, and spirit.

Before I wanted to be an actor, I aspired to become a doctor. Once, I played a doctor in a movie when I switched brains with comedian Dudley Moore in "Like Father Like Son." While it can be funny when actors pretend to be doctors, it's never funny when doctors turn out to be actors. The COVID pandemic removed the masks and revealed the true physicians from the paid imposters. Dr. Barke turned out to be the real deal, putting his patients before profits and valuing health over hype. Dr. Barke is not only intelligent and knowledgeable but also compassionate, an excellent communicator, a lover of fine cigars, and committed to telling his patients the unvarnished truth about their health and wellness when "fake news" and "disinformation" abounds.

I first met Dr. Barke at church when I picked up a very helpful booklet called "XYZ." "I wish I could find a doctor like this author," I thought to myself. Then I did; he was standing right next to me! We became friends. At Christmas time, he got me into the best kind of trouble - his courage helped me set thousands free from the FEAR virus by inviting willing families to wholesome Christmas carol singalongs at the beach at sunset. After nine months of California lockdowns, many of us felt trapped, and the chance to breathe fresh air, expand our lungs, and reconnect with family and friends had us all singing with full voice, "Joy to the World!" Dr. Barke's famous YouTube video explaining the limitations of PPEs to protect us from viruses and then revealing his own preferred piece of Personal Protection Equipment got me thinking, "This doc is for me!"

His practice is state of the art, and his strategies exemplify the principles of the Hippocratic Oath: to prescribe only beneficial treatments, according to the doctor's abilities and judgment; to refrain from causing harm or hurt; and to live an exemplary personal and professional life.

I hope this book helps you start your days out right, setting the tone and pace for a healthy outlook through a collection of proven health tips, inspiring Bible passages, and memorable quotes that will bring health to your body, strength to your bones, warmth to your heart, and clarity to your mind. Better than chicken soup, these morning meditations will also nourish your soul.

"A joyful heart is good medicine, but a broken spirit dries up the bones." (Proverbs 17:22)

For these reasons, I highly recommend you read Dr. Barke's Morning Message as part of your daily wellness routine. You'll be thankful you did!

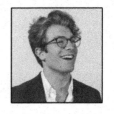

Forward Written by Will Witt

Bestselling Author of "How to Win Friends and Influence Enemies".

Modernity would make us believe that we are living in the most technologically, medically, and factually advanced society in all of humanity's history. We are told that we are at the apex of innovation, and soon enough, we will be able to modify and "enhance" our bodies and minds in ways only previously thought of in science fiction novels and movies. Yet, despite this, our world is becoming unhealthier, our people are getting fatter, and many suffer from ailments of the mind at unprecedented levels never before seen.

Medicine in America has become nothing more than "pay for play." Many doctors prescribe drugs for their own benefit and the lining of their pockets. Universities research issues funded by the biggest donors, and big pharma takes advantage of the American people whenever they get a chance. Nutritionists peddle unhealthy practices designed by bogus government health standards. Everywhere you look, it seems like nobody is preaching the true, good, and moral healthy lifestyles needed for a strong and happy population.

Dr. Jeff Barke is the antithesis of the modern medical lexicon. Dr. Barke has researched and sought out the best medical and health information available. He preaches an approach that is less reliant on pills and medicine but focuses on food and lifestyle. Dr. Barke puts the patient first, not profits.
Dr. Barke gets it.

As my doctor, Dr. Barke has always been upfront about my health and has never shied away from telling me the hard truth about what I needed. Instead of just prescribing me a pill, Dr. Barke worked personally with me on a plan to not just band-aid the problem but fix the problem. His wealth of knowledge about health and medicine along with his integrity have made Dr. Barke my most trusted advisor for any questions about health and wellness.

This book will give you the tools to live a healthy lifestyle, not just patches to avoid the problems you may already have, but real answers on how to tackle your ailments and flourish with your health. Where other health professionals give boilerplate responses and platitudes, Dr. Barke provides you with the hard truth on how to really fix and prevent any maladies you may have.

Many things he presents in this book may be difficult, and it may be hard to implement all the lifestyle changes he advises, but I promise you, the hard way is the better way, and you will thank yourself for years to come if you follow the ideas and facts within this work.

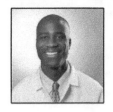

Forward Written by Dr. Joseph Ladapo

Author of "Transcend Fear: A Blueprint for Mindful Leadership in Public Health," Professor, University of Florida College of Medicine, and Surgeon General of Florida.

The reason so many people admire Dr. Barke is that, despite being a successful and highly sought-after doctor, he remains humble, kind, and genuinely caring. The reason I hold him in high regard is due to his courage and unwavering commitment to speaking his truth. In his new book, "Morning Message," Dr. Barke identifies the core components of health, such as physical activity, exposure to sunlight, and consumption of nutritious, wholesome food.

He dispels many of the health myths that have taken root in our minds as a result of industrial greed and disconnection from our relationship with God and nature. The time has come for all of us to reestablish that connection, and Dr. Barke illuminates the path.

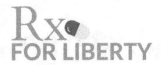

Morning Message

Priorities

We get hung up too often on the material things that are not important, when we should be focused on the eternal.

That is, relationships with family, our prayer and meditation life, and taking care of ourselves. Truly focus on things that elevate us, and not just things that are material in nature.

Morning Message

If your doctor tells you:

Avoid eggs
Avoid the sun
Eat less meat
Eat fake meat
Go on a low salt diet
Raw dairy is dangerous

It's time to get a new doctor!

Morning Message

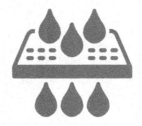

Benefits of Drinking Purified Water

Healthier skin
More energy
Assists digestion & internal functions
Rids harmful contaminants
Never drink tap water (government water)

Morning Message

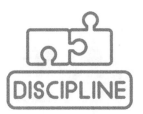

The price of discipline

Think clean eating is expensive?
Try the cost of illness.
Think weight lifting is dangerous?
Try being weak.
Think fitness is time consuming?
Try waiting in the ER.
Think meditation is a waste of time?
Try chronic stress and illness.

Discipline brings freedom, independence, and optimal health.

Morning Message

"The time to repair the roof is when the sun is shining."

-John F. Kennedy

Don't wait for illness to improve your health. Your daily choices create habits.

Your habits determine your future.

Morning Message
OPTIMAL HEALTH
Weekend Commitments

Physical Health:

Take a 30-minute walk today

Go to bed early tonight

Spiritual Health:

Attend a spiritual or mindfullness workshop

Tell a friend about your experience

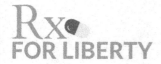

Morning Message

Foster Healthy Breathing

Habits: Practice diaphragmatic breathing techniques to promote deep, mindful breathing and to enhance oxygenation.

Morning Message

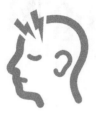

Headache Remedy

Hydrate!
Cold compresses!
Neck stretches!
Sleep!
Warm Epson salt bath!
Meditate!
No drugs needed!

Morning Message

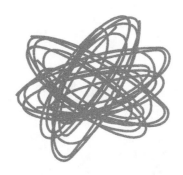

Embrace a Minimalist Lifestyle

Simplify your living space, and let go of
unnecessary possessions to create a
clutter-free environment that promotes
calmness and clarity.

Morning Message

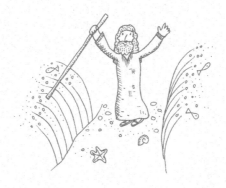

Faith > Fear

Moses took the first step, THEN the Red Sea parted. He trusted the plan. Take the first step! Don't be paralyzed by fear.

Morning Message

Give your sorrows to the Lord and find peace in His love. We are praying for you to have comfort and feel His grace in your life every day.

Morning Message
OPTIMAL HEALTH
Write down your own commitments

Physical Health:

_____
_____
_____
_____
_____
_____
_____
_____

Spiritual Health:

_____
_____
_____
_____
_____
_____
_____
_____

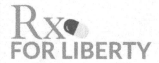

Morning Message

Preventing Heart Disease

It is not about cholesterol or saturated fat, rather it is about inflammation and metabolic dysfunction. Eat clean, get daily sunshine, and manage your stress.

Morning Message

My Favorite Supplements

Sunshine
Exercise
Coffee with raw goat milk & cinnamon
Manuka honey
Hugs
Connection
A purring cat

Morning Message

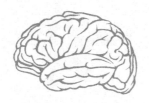

Radical Health

While genetics are important, how we take care of ourselves is far more determinative. Most illness, including physical and mental, is self-inflicted.

Seek radical health by becoming literate about your body, mind, and soul.

Morning Message

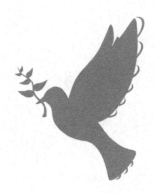

Health care and health is not something that comes naturally. We need to learn and fight to understand how to take care of ourselves – our physical, mental, and spiritual health.

Morning Message

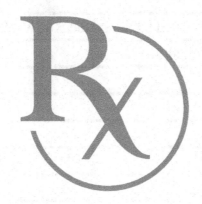

Medical Freedom

We need to teach ourselves about medical freedom and liberty. Take control of your own health.

Morning Message
OPTIMAL HEALTH
Weekend Commitments

Physical Health:

Cut down on processed foods and focus on whole foods

Cut down on drinking alcohol

_____

_____

_____

_____

_____

Spiritual Health:

Prayer and meditation

Attend a sermon or view it online

_____

_____

_____

_____

_____

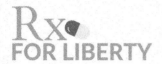
FOR LIBERTY

Morning Message

Wellness is the complete integration of body, mind, and soul–the realization that everything we do, think, feel, and believe has an effect on our state of well-being.

Morning Message

Don't Worry

Don't worry about anything. Tell God what you need, and thank Him for all He has done, then you will experience God's peace, which exceeds anything that we can understand.

Morning Message

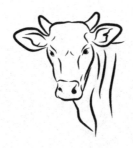

Common Lies

Just a little chlorine in your water is fine. It kills the bacteria.

The neurotoxin fluoride in your water is within government standards, nothing to worry about.

The Dept. of Agriculture will allow mRNA vaccines in cattle. Trust us, it's safe and effective.

Morning Message

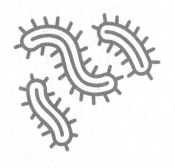

The Gut Microbiome

What we feed our gut either supports our health or fans the flames of inflammation, and sometimes we don't know which will happen.

There is wonderful food sensitivity and allergy testing. Both US Biotech or Alcat are available commercially to help you decipher how what you are eating is effecting your body.

Morning Message

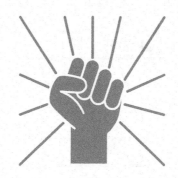

I can do all things through
Christ which strengthens me.
-Philippians 4:13

Morning Message
OPTIMAL HEALTH
Weekend Commitments

Physical Health:

Drink more water

Cut down on drinking alcohol

_____

_____

_____

_____

Spiritual Health:

Restart a meditation program

Pray daily

_____

_____

_____

_____

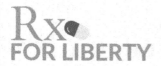

Morning Message

EMF (Electro Magnetic Fields)
can destroy and damage our DNA,
increase our cancer risk, disrupt
our sleep, cause headaches,
dizziness, hormonal imbalance,
and immune system problems.

Use wired headphones only.
Limit cell-phone usage.
Turn wifi off at night.

Morning Message

z^z**Z**

Sleep supplements

Melatonin
Magnesium
Valerian Root
GABA
Ashwagandha

Morning Message

Benefits of Morning Sunshine

Production of Vitamin D
Enhances mood and mental health
Reduces inflammation
Enhances melatonin production
Boosts immune function
Improves cardiovascular health
Improves bone health
Boosts overall well-being
Helps with the sleep/wake cycle

It's still free!

Morning Message

Side Effects of Eating Clean

More energy
Increased libido
Mental clarity
Reduced risk of heart disease
Reduced risk of cancer
Reduced risk of diabetes
Reduced anxiety/depression
Increased longevity

Morning Message

Embrace Joy and Laughter

Seek out experiences that bring you joy. Surround yourself with humor and allow yourself to laugh freely to uplift your spirit.

Morning Message
OPTIMAL HEALTH
Weekend Commitments

Physical Health:

Eat healthy

Exercise a few days a week

Spiritual Health:

Practice positive self talk

Take time to practice gratitude

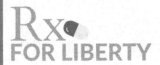

FOR LIBERTY

Morning Message

"It is one of the most beautiful
compensations in life that no man
can sincerely try to help another
without helping himself."

-Ralph Waldo Emerson

Morning Message

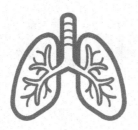

**One of my favorite supplements:
Organ Synergy by
Designs for Health**

Whole Foods equivalent of a multivitamin
Grass-fed, organic beef organs from New Zealand
Liver, heart, kidney, and pancreas
Loaded with vitamins and minerals
Nutrient-dense
Family owned company
Glass bottles

Morning Message

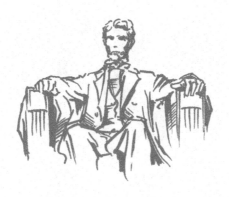

"In the end, it's not the years in your life that count. It's the life in your years."

-Abraham Lincoln

Morning Message

In the stillness of your heart lies the wisdom to guide you on your radical journey toward optimal health of the mind, body, and soul.

Morning Message

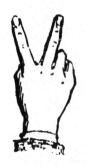

Self Talk

By far, one of the most significant stresses on our mind is caused by how we speak to ourselves. The loudest and most frequent voice we hear is our self-talk. Learn to control your self-talk, and you'll be on your way to peace.

Morning Message
OPTIMAL HEALTH
Write down your own commitments

Physical Health:

_____

_____

_____

_____

_____

_____

_____

_____

Spiritual Health:

_____

_____

_____

_____

_____

_____

_____

_____

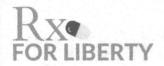

Rx *●*
FOR LIBERTY

Morning Message

Anxiety Remedies

Exercise
Meditation
Morning sunshine
Deep breathing
Support from friends and family

Supplements: Ashwagandha
Magnesium, Fish-Oil, GABA, and
L-Theanine

Trust God + Chill

Morning Message

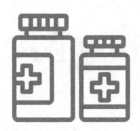

Big Pharma is the problem, not the solution: Ozempic, Mounjaro, Rybelsus

GLP-1 (glucagon-like-peptide-1) drugs

Tricks your body to think it's full
Tells your pancreas to produce more insulin
Stops your liver from releasing stored glucose
No long-term safety studies
Potential serious side effects
Does not alter behavior or habits
Very expensive

Instead: Do the hard work to eat clean, reduce stress, get sunshine, and hydrate with purified water.

Morning Message

The day ahead holds one million possibilities for us to trust God and to respond with strength that is not our own; will we surrender so He can usher us into victory?

Morning Message

Allergy Prevention

Overreaction to a foreign substance causes IgE antibody production which binds to mast-cells which then release histamine. Itching may differentiate allergies from infection.

Always check with your own doctor before getting treatment.

Morning Message

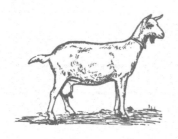

Why Goat Milk?

Higher protein content
Easier to digest
Loaded with healthy probiotics
More nutritious than cow's milk
Good for your skin
Prevents insulin resistance
Tastes delicious
Less lactose

Morning Message
OPTIMAL HEALTH
Weekend Commitments

Physical Health:

Try goat milk

Look into a new supplement

Spiritual Health:

Journal your thoughts

Tell someone about your journey

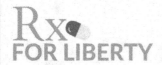

FOR LIBERTY

Morning Message

Embrace the power of
gratitude, and watch as your
life transforms. For it is
through gratitude that we
invite abundance and joy
into our lives.

Morning Message

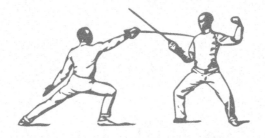

Choose kindness as your compass,
for it is the language that
transcends all barriers
and unites humanity.

Morning Message

Detoxification

Dilution is the solution to pollution...
drink lots of purified water!

Sweating
Epsom salt baths
Daily bowel movements
Exercise to circulate your blood
Daily sunshine

Morning Message

True medical freedom is being in charge of your own health, relying on your God-given immune system and not relying on the pharmaceutical industry.

Support your immune system with clean eating, a reliance on God, and a deep devotion to lifelong learning.

Morning Message

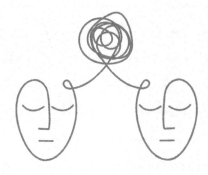

A deep human connection is
necessary for optimal health –
there is no substitute.

Morning Message
OPTIMAL HEALTH
Weekend Commitments

Physical Health:

Drink less soda

Drink more water

_____

_____

_____

_____

Spiritual Health:

Pray for a friend today

Embody your higher self

_____

_____

_____

_____

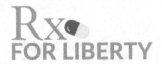

Rx
FOR LIBERTY

Morning Message

Tips to Maximize Focus

Prayer

Eat healthy

Avoid sugar

Daily exercise

Daily sunshine

Meditation

Fish Oil supplements

Morning Message

Want to transform your health?

Drink 64 oz purified water daily
Get 10-15 min of sunshine daily
Walk for an hour a day
Lift weights 3-4 days per week
Meditate/pray daily
Get >7 hours of sleep per night
Eliminate refined sugar
Eliminate inflammatory oils
Give love to your pet/companion!

Morning Message

Happiness

It's a choice that we make on a daily basis. It's not an external thing, it's an internal thing. It is a result of our actions that create desired feelings. If we act a certain way, the feelings will follow.

Morning Message

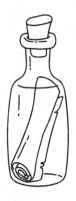

Too often when we are in pain, we immediately look for a prescription or an over the counter product to make our pain go away. Listen to your body, pain can be a message.

Morning Message

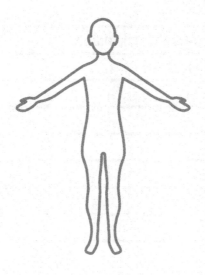

Take care of your body. It's the only place you have to live. - Jim Rohn

Morning Message
OPTIMAL HEALTH
Weekend Commitments

Physical Health:

Use a reusable water to track intake

Eat whole nutritious food

_____

_____

_____

_____

_____

Spiritual Health:

Practice mindfulness

Start a new book

_____

_____

_____

_____

_____

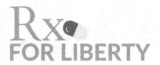

Morning Message

Cinnamon

Cinnamon is a very healthy spice, the second most popular spice in the United States.

It has anti-inflammatory, anti-bacterial, and antioxidant properties. It can also help regulate blood glucose and reduce the risk of blood clotting.

Morning Message

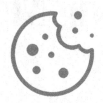

Cookies sold by girls in uniform

High fructose corn syrup
Processed vegetable oil
Refined sugar
Food dyes
Preservatives
Artificial flavors

Not healthy... but so delicious

Morning Message

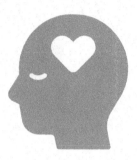

Benefits of Fasting

Autophagy–cellular regeneration and repair
Decreased insulin resistance
Metabolic resiliency and flexibility
Mental clarity
Improved immune system
Saves on grocery bills

Morning Message

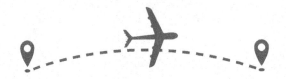

Flying Smarter

Never restrict your breathing with a mask.
Hydrate before, during, and after the flight.
Avoid airline-provided food or snacks–it is garbage!
Bring your own nutrient-rich food.
Avoid sugar and don't hate me... alcohol!

Morning Message

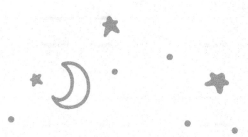

Trust Your Intuition

Cultivate a deeper connection with your inner wisdom and intuition. Learn to trust God. Make choices that align with His will to your authentic self.

Morning Message
OPTIMAL HEALTH
Weekend Commitments

Physical Health:

Consider a fast (consult with your doctor)

Food log your meals for the day

Spiritual Health:

Send an inspirational message to someone

Do some deep breathing and sit with your thoughts

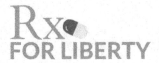

Morning Message

Finding Your Purpose

Being in nature is helpful to review our own purpose.

For me, it's when I'm deeply connected with people and feel I'm making a positive change in peoples' lives.

Do something to make a difference.

Morning Message

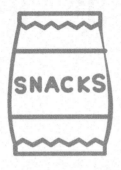

Healthy Snacks

Fruit and veggies
Grass-fed organic cottage cheese
Paleovalley Superfood Bar
Grass-fed beef stick
Raw nuts/seeds
Hard boiled pasture raised egg
Yogurt with Manuka honey

Morning Message

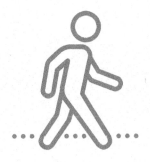

Hypertension = High Blood Pressure

Natural Remedies:
Reduce stress with meditation
Lose weight
Daily movement
Drink plenty of purified water
Magnesium supplements
Grape seed extract
Daily sunshine

Morning Message

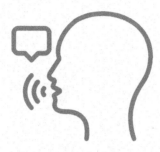

Speak Positive Affirmations:

Who will you be in 5 years?
I am_____

How will you feel to be this person?
I will feel_____

What goals will you accomplish?
I accomplished_____

Morning Message

The Lord walks beside us through the darkness and leads us back to peace.

Even though I walk through the darkest valley, I will fear no evil, for you are with me; your rod and your staff, they comfort me. Psalm 23:4

Morning Message
OPTIMAL HEALTH
Write down your own commitments

Physical Health:

_____
_____
_____
_____
_____
_____
_____
_____

Spiritual Health:

_____
_____
_____
_____
_____
_____
_____
_____

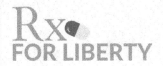

Morning Message

Exercise should be a celebration of
what you can accomplish, not a
consequence of your poor
nutrition choice.

Morning Message

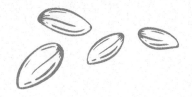

Prioritize Omega-3 Fatty Acids for Brain Health and Inflammation Reduction

Fatty fish
Fish-oil
Cod-liver oil
Nuts and seeds

Morning Message

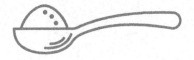

Sugar = Inflammation

Read the labels, it's in everything.
Artificial sugars are also bad,
even the ones you are told are okay.
Need something sweet? Try some raw honey!

Morning Message

Optimal Health

The path to optimal health begins with nurturing your soul, for it is the foundation upon which all aspects of your well-being are built.

Morning Message

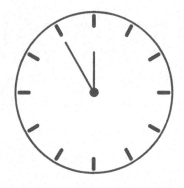

If you don't make time for your wellness, you will
be forced to make time for your illness.
Read that again.

Morning Message
OPTIMAL HEALTH
Weekend Commitments

Physical Health:

Say NO to an unhealthy junk food

Increase your water intake if you're not properly hydrated

_____

_____

_____

_____

_____

Spiritual Health:

Speak life into your body

Practice mindfulness this week

_____

_____

_____

_____

_____

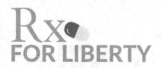
Morning Message

Hydrate with Herbal Teas

Drink herbal teas like chamomile, peppermint, or ginger to stay hydrated while enjoying their potential health benefits.

Morning Message

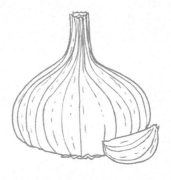

Spice it Up

Incorporate herbs and spices like turmeric, ginger, garlic, cinnamon, and rosemary to enhance flavor while providing antioxidants and anti-inflammatory effects.

Morning Message

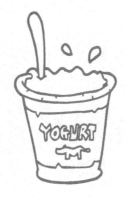

Fermented foods can improve gut health

Include fermented foods like yogurt, kefir, sauerkraut, kimchi, and kombucha to support gut health and improve digestion.

Morning Message

Cast all your anxiety on
Him because He cares for you.

1 Peter 5:7

Morning Message

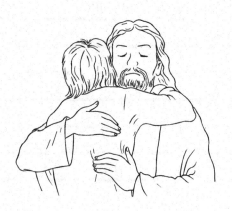

True faith means holding nothing back. It means putting every hope in God's fidelity to His Promises.

Morning Message
OPTIMAL HEALTH
Weekend Commitments

Physical Health:

Try a new tea

Cook a meal in, instead of eating out

Spiritual Health:

Attend or listen to a service

Compliment a stranger

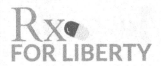
FOR LIBERTY

Morning Message

Cook at Home

Prepare meals at home using fresh, whole ingredients to have more control over the quality and nutritional content of your meals.

Morning Message

Embrace the beauty of imperfection, for it is through our struggles and challenges that we find strength, growth, and profound transformation.

Morning Message

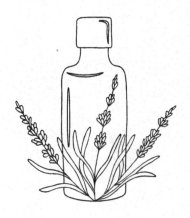

Explore Essential Oils

Use essential oils like lavender, eucalyptus, or tea tree oil for aromatherapy, relaxation, or as natural remedies for minor ailments.

Morning Message

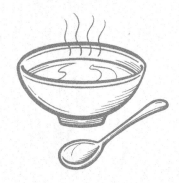

Incorporate Bone Broth

Prepare homemade bone broth using organic, grass-fed bones to support joint health, digestion, and immune function.

Morning Message

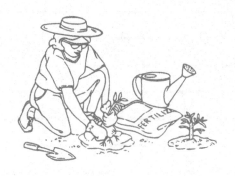

Trust in the LORD with all your heart, and do not lean on your own understanding. In all your ways acknowledge Him, and He will make straight your paths.

Romans 15:13

Morning Message
OPTIMAL HEALTH
Weekend Commitments

Physical Health:

Drink more water

Cut down on drinking sugar

Spiritual Health:

Restart a meditation

Pray every morning

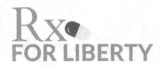

Morning Message

The Holy Spirit calls us to change, then gives us the power and strength to overcome all obstacles.

Morning Message

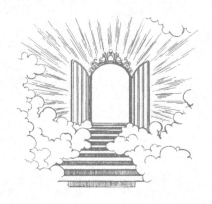

"Health is a state of complete harmony of the body, mind, and spirit. When one is free from physical disabilities and mental distractions, the gates of the soul open."
- B.K.S. Iyengar

Morning Message

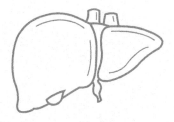

Support Liver Health

Include liver supportive foods like leafy greens, beets, artichokes, and dandelion root tea to promote detoxification and better overall liver function.

Morning Message

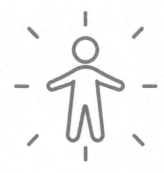

Optimal health is not a destination, but a continuous journey of self-discovery, growth, and transformation.

Morning Message

Be strong! Be fearless! Don't be afraid and don't be scared by your enemies, because the Lord your God is the one who marches with you. He won't let you down, and he won't abandon you.

Deuteronomy 31:6

Morning Message
OPTIMAL HEALTH
Weekend Commitments

Physical Health:

Stretch or do yoga

Go to bed earlier

_____

_____

_____

_____

_____

Spiritual Health:

Journal a prayer

Believe things will get better

_____

_____

_____

_____

_____

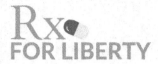

Morning Message

Try Herbal Steam Inhalations

Use herbal steam inhalations with eucalyptus, peppermint, or chamomile to relieve congestion and promote respiratory health.

Morning Message

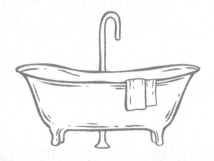

Use Epsom Salt Baths

Enjoy a warm bath with Epsom salts to relax muscles, reduce stress, and promote detoxification.

Morning Message

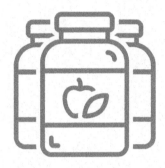

Consider Nutritional Supplements

Discuss with a healthcare professional the potential benefits of nutritional supplements like Vitamin D, Magnesium, and Omega-3 Fatty Acids to address specific deficiencies or support overall health.

Morning Message

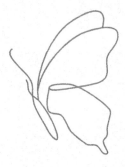

Find peace in the present moment, for it is
the gateway to eternal serenity and
profound inner transformation.

Morning Message

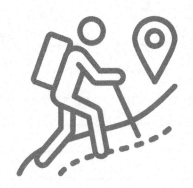

God didn't give us a spirit that is timid, but one that is powerful, loving, and self-controlled.

Timothy 1:7

Morning Message
OPTIMAL HEALTH
Weekend Commitments

Physical Health:

Try a new vegetable

Sign up for an exercise class (if physically able)

Spiritual Health:

Say a prayer

Send a prayer

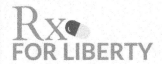

Morning Message

"Happiness is not something ready-made. It comes from your own actions." - Dalai Lama

Morning Message

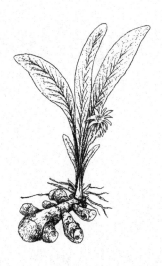

Turmeric

Incorporate turmeric, a natural anti-inflammatory spice, in cooking or as a supplement to potentially alleviate inflammation-related conditions.

Morning Message

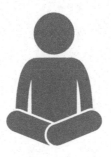

Do not be anxious about anything, but in every situation, by prayer and petition, with thanksgiving, present your requests to God.

Philippians 4:6

Morning Message

Mental Clarity and Focus

Discover activities that bring you mental clarity and focus. Explore practices such as meditation, journaling, and brain-training exercises to enhance your cognitive abilities and support mental well-being.

Morning Message

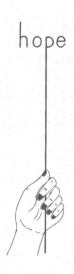

Endurance produces character, and character produces hope. This hope doesn't put us to shame, because the love of God has been poured out in our hearts through the Holy Spirit, who has been given to us.

Romans 5:4-5

Morning Message
OPTIMAL HEALTH
Weekend Commitments

Physical Health:

Do some grounding in nature/outside

Spend some time meal planning/prepping

Spiritual Health:

Think positive thoughts

Read a chapter in your new book

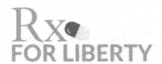

Morning Message

Holistic Healing

Explore holistic approaches to healing. Research integrative medicine approaches that combine conventional and alternative therapies to address your specific health concerns and support your overall well-being.

Morning Message

Love Yourself!

Practice self-acceptance and self-love.
Embrace your unique qualities and attributes,
celebrating your individuality and nurturing
a positive self-image.

Morning Message

Every step you take on your journey is a sacred act of self-discovery. Embrace each experience with gratitude and openness.

Morning Message

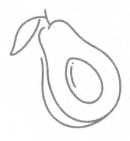

Superfoods

Pasture raised eggs
Organic blueberries
Raw dairy
Raw honey
Grass-fed organic beef

Morning Message

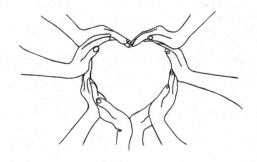

Examine me, Lord; put me to the test! Purify my mind and my heart. Because your faithful love is right in front of me — I walk in your truth! I don't spend time with people up to no good; I don't keep company with liars.

Psalm 26:2-4

Morning Message
OPTIMAL HEALTH
Weekend Commitments

Physical Health:

Give yourself grace on your journey

Cut down on eating processed food

_____

_____

_____

_____

Spiritual Health:

Connect with like-minded people

Engage in mindfullness

_____

_____

_____

_____

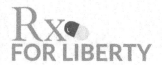

FOR LIBERTY

Morning Message

Dopamine

The pleasure/satisfaction/motivation
chemical in our brain.

Here's how to increase your
dopamine levels:

Proper sleep
Exercise
Eat healthy
Listen to your favorite music
Sunshine

Morning Message

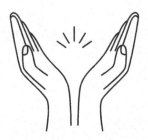

Gratitude

I am grateful to God for His abundance and forgiveness.

I am grateful to those that allow me to be part of their journey.

I am grateful for the grace and kindness of my friends and family!

I am grateful for my health and my God-given immune system!

I am grateful for those that teach me how to be a better doctor and a better person!

Morning Message

Radical Health

1 out of 5 children are obese.
50% are overweight.

It's time for your radical change.

Clean eating, purified water, daily
sunshine, meditation, and exercise.

That is Radical Health.

Morning Message

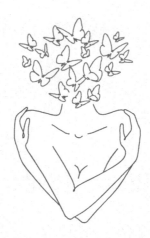

Unveil the hidden treasures within your heart and unleash the boundless love that resides within you. It is the essence of your true nature.

Morning Message

But Jesus looked at them and said, 'with man this is impossible, but with God all things are possible.'

Matthew 19:26

Morning Message
OPTIMAL HEALTH
Write down your own commitments

Physical Health:

_____

_____

_____

_____

_____

_____

_____

Spiritual Health:

_____

_____

_____

_____

_____

_____

_____

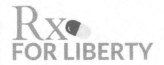

FOR LIBERTY

Morning Message

Incorporate adaptogenic herbs, like Ashwagandha or Rhodiola, to support your body's resilience to stress.

Morning Message

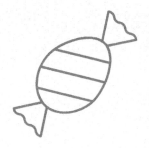

Watch your food - read the labels

Red Dye #40
Yellow Dye #5 & #6
Refined sugar
Vegetable oils
Artificial sweeteners

Morning Message

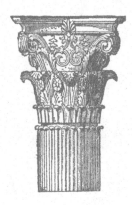

Therefore, my beloved brothers, be steadfast, immovable, always abounding in the work of the Lord, knowing that in the Lord your labor is not in vain.

1 Corinthians 15:58

Morning Message

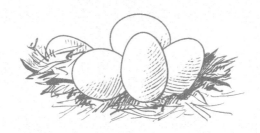

Pasture Raised Eggs = Superfood

Despite the constant back and forth about eggs and health, it's a myth that eggs are bad for you. They have minimal effect on blood cholesterol in the majority of people, and they're a great source of protein and nutrients.

Morning Message

Gratitude is showing appreciation or thankfulness to someone. Take a second today to show your love, support, and thanks to the people around you.

Morning Message
OPTIMAL HEALTH
Weekend Commitments

Physical Health:

Toss foods or donate junk food

Avoid inflammatory oils

Spiritual Health:

Journal about your current emotions

Meet up with a friend and fellowship

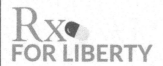

FOR LIBERTY

Morning Message

Your breath is a bridge
between the physical and the
spiritual realms. Honor its
divine dance and find
tranquility in the present.

Morning Message

Optimal Health

Focusing on optimal health, not weight loss, will create the best version of you. Focusing on spiritual and emotional health, not status or popularity, will create a path to happiness.

Morning Message

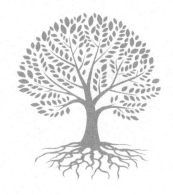

Habits

You either need to change your vision or change your habits. Optimal health requires optimal habits. This includes emotional and spiritual health. You can't get healthy with the same habits that created your current state.

Morning Message

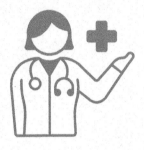

Most physicians do not have the time or knowledge to teach patients how to optimize their health. Find a doctor that does, or you are wasting your time and money.

Morning Message

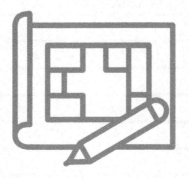

'For I know the plans I have for you,'
declares the Lord, 'plans to prosper you
and not to harm you, plans to give you
hope and a future.'

Jeremiah 29:11

Morning Message
OPTIMAL HEALTH
Weekend Commitments

Physical Health:

Try a new healthy recipe

Brew some fresh tea or kombucha

Spiritual Health:

Take a walk in nature

Listen to an uplifting song

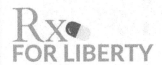

Morning Message

Genetics

Your genes load the gun, but your lifestyle pulls the trigger. Fix your lifestyle if you want to achieve optimal health. Stop blaming your genetics.

Morning Message

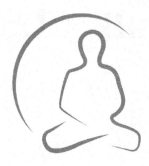

Equanimity

Evenness of mind, especially under stress. Meditation can improve sleep, reduce anxiety, and depression.

Morning Message

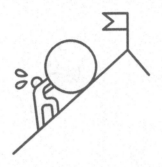

Have faith in God, for truly I tell you, if you have faith as small as a mustard seed, you can say to this mountain, 'Move from here to there,' and it will move. Nothing will be impossible for you.

Matthew 17:20

Morning Message

An Apple a Day

Yes, it's an actual thing!
Apples are loaded with
anti-inflammatory polyphenols.
Great for gut health and loaded
with fiber.

Morning Message

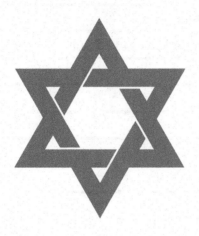

Trust in the Lord with all your heart and lean not on your own understanding; in all your ways submit to Him, and He will make your paths straight.

Proverbs 3:5-6

Morning Message
OPTIMAL HEALTH
Weekend Commitments

Physical Health:

Track your water intake

Experiment with new spices like turmeric

Spiritual Health:

Do an act of kindness

Get enough sleep

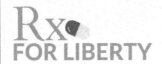
FOR LIBERTY

Morning Message

Practice Mindful Eating

Pay attention to your food choices, eat slowly, and savor each bite to foster a deeper connection with your body's nutritional needs.

Morning Message

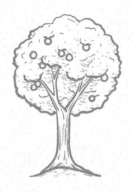

Prioritize Whole Foods

Consume a balanced diet rich in fruits, vegetables, whole grains, lean proteins, and healthy fats to provide essential nutrients for your body.

Morning Message

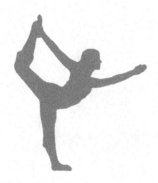

Get Regular Exercise

Engage in physical activity that you enjoy, such as walking, jogging, yoga, or dancing to enhance cardiovascular health, flexibility, and overall fitness.

Morning Message

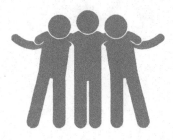

Foster Positive Relationships

Surround yourself with supportive, uplifting individuals who encourage personal growth and provide a sense of community.

Morning Message

Fight the good fight of the faith.
Take hold of the eternal life to which
you were called when you made
your good confession in the presence
of many witnesses.

1 Timothy 6:12

Morning Message
OPTIMAL HEALTH
Weekend Commitments

Physical Health:

Set reminders to eat healthy meals

Make new healthy habits

_____

_____

_____

_____

Spiritual Health:

Connect in nature

Self reflection

_____

_____

_____

_____

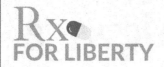

Rx
FOR LIBERTY

Morning Message

Practice Gratitude

Take a few moments each day to appreciate the blessings in your life and cultivate a positive mindset.

Morning Message

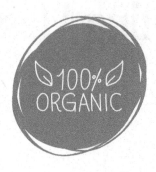

Limit Toxins

Reduce exposure to environmental toxins by opting for organic foods, using natural cleaning and personal care products, and minimizing the use of plastics.

Morning Message

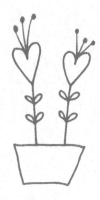

Compassion

Cultivate a heart full of compassion, and you will illuminate the world with your kindness, empathy, and healing presence.

Morning Message

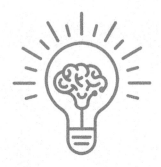

Practice Self-Care

Set aside time for activities that bring you joy and relaxation, whether it's reading, taking baths, listening to music, or pursuing creative hobbies.

Morning Message

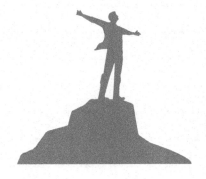

Now faith is confidence in what we hope for and assurance about what we do not see.

Hebrews 11:1

Morning Message
OPTIMAL HEALTH
Weekend Commitments

Physical Health:

Set specific times to workout or stretch

Gradually replace soda with water

Spiritual Health:

Deepen your understanding with faith

Seek guidance from a mentor if needed

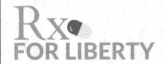

Morning Message

Engage in Lifelong Learning

Challenge your mind by exploring
new interests, acquiring
knowledge, and engaging in
stimulating activities to promote
cognitive vitality.

Morning Message

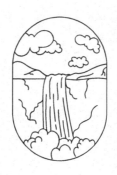

Water

60% to 70% of our body is made up of water, and most of us don't drink enough of it.

Purified drinking water improves our mental performance, helps with weight loss, increases our mood and flushes toxins away.

Morning Message

Connect with Community

Engage in meaningful ways with your local community; volunteer or participate in group activities that align with your values.

Morning Message

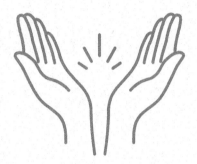

Foster a Spiritual Connection

Explore practices like meditation, prayer, or connecting with a higher power to nurture your soul and deepen your sense of purpose.

Morning Message

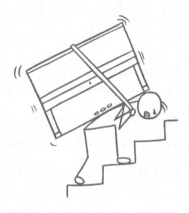

Trust in the Lord with all your heart, and do not lean on your own understanding. In all your ways acknowledge Him, and he will make straight your paths.

Proverbs 3:5-6

Morning Message
OPTIMAL HEALTH
Write down your own commitments

Physical Health:

_____

_____

_____

_____

_____

_____

_____

Spiritual Health:

_____

_____

_____

_____

_____

_____

_____

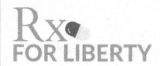

Morning Message

Popcorn!

Avoid microwave popcorn, it's not good for you. It is filled with PFAs (Polyfluoroalkyl Substances), and often contains inflammatory seed and vegetable oils.

Anytime you super heat plastic, it releases toxic chemicals into your food.

Try popping corn on the stove with avocado oil, organic butter, or ghee.

Morning Message

Stay clear of Antibiotics when possible

They have a role to play, but should be very limited, as they can cause unintended consequences like gut dysbiosis. Antibiotics kill indiscriminately and can cause antibiotic resistance. Avoid them, except in extreme circumstances.

Morning Message

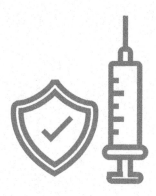

Ouchy Arm Thingy

Informed consent is best when considering any vaccine for yourself or loved ones.

1. What are the risks?
2. What are the side effects?
3. What are the ingredients?

Morning Message

Self-Awareness

Pay attention to your body's cues and responses. Develop a deeper awareness of your body's signals and responses, such as hunger, fatigue, or discomfort, and respond with self-care and self-compassion.

Morning Message

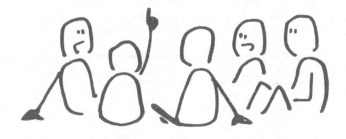

Therefore, my dear brothers and sisters,
stand firm. Let nothing move you. Always
give yourselves fully to the work of the Lord,
because you know that your labor in the
Lord is not in vain.

1 Corinthians 15:58

Morning Message
OPTIMAL HEALTH
Weekend Commitments

Physical Health:

Listen to your body and what it needs

Treat yourself with something you enjoy

Spiritual Health:

Set intentions for the next week

express your spirituality through art, music, writing, etc.

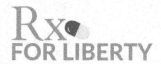

Morning Message

Create a Peaceful Environment

Design your living space to promote tranquility and peace, incorporating elements like plants, natural lighting, and soothing colors.

Morning Message

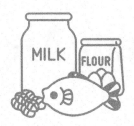

Standard Diet

Processed foods with dyes and preservatives
Refined sugar
Antibiotic/hormone-infused, grain-fed meat
Vegetable/seed oil added food
Tap water

Holistic Health Diet

Grass-fed organic meat
No refined sugar
Raw dairy
Pasture raised eggs
Raw honey
Purified water

Morning Message

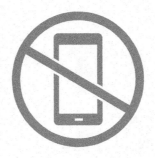

Engage in Digital Detox

Take regular breaks from technology. Set boundaries around screen time to reduce mental clutter and to promote presence.

Morning Message

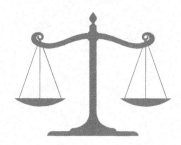

Create a Balanced Lifestyle

Strive for a balance between work, leisure, social connections, and personal time, ensuring that all aspects of your life are nurtured.

Morning Message

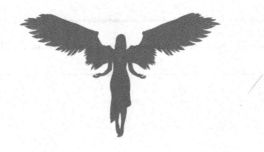

Rise up... take courage and do it.

Ezra 10:4

Morning Message
OPTIMAL HEALTH
Write which changes you've made

Physical Health:

_____

_____

_____

_____

_____

_____

_____

_____

Spiritual Health:

_____

_____

_____

_____

_____

_____

_____

_____

"So blessed to have found your page. I enjoy your Morning Messages! I might need to come see you soon.. Have a great day!" -**Mervat**

"Love following you and all the awesome info you provide. Thank you for your service" -**Farnaz**

"My name is Debbie. I am 49, mother of 3 boys who used to play travel hockey. I live in Central California and have been teaching elementary for 25 years. I started following the Frontline doctors when the chaos started and have appreciated the natural approaches to healthcare." -**Debbie**

"So happy to have connected with you Dr. Barke! You are a rare find in the medical field and a great example of how not all Drs are created equally. Keep spreading your wisdom and fighting the good fight!" -**Natalie**

@RxforLiberty
Instagram Testimonies

"Impressive! Started following you in 2020 right after I retired from teaching and the sh*t hit the fan...enjoy following you." -**Kim**

"Thank you for your service to our country. And God bless you for the way you are practicing medicine... you are a rare breed, & I'm grateful for you." -**Sharon**

"Thank you Dr. Barke for what you do. You are such a blessing. I look forward to your morning messages and I've learned so much from you. I'm a dentist in a small town and I own my own practice. I could not do this without my husband, the man that I prayed for many years. I was a pediatric nurse in the icu, burn unit and critical care transport. I want to thank you for your service in the military and also for your daily inspiration to all of us." -**Annie**

"Thank you for all you do! I'm a mom that co-created PragerUkids.com.. so we can raise kids with love and appreciation for America." -**Jill**

"A voice of sound, non biased reason...a real encouragement of common sense during the plague" -**Rob**

"Someone I would be proud to call my Doc! And feel completely SAFE with my Health and Wellness! Thanks for what you've been doing to educate the completely Ignorant!" -**Julia**

"Tangie, a mom of 4 out here in Arizona. You caught my attention in 2020 and you are one of the heroes who equipped my husband and I to keep our family safe and informed during all the insanity. We are forever grateful. Thanks for taking your oath seriously. You're a gem." **Anonymous**

"I always look forward to your morning messages and have learned so much! Thank you for all that you do!" -**Erin**

@RxforLiberty
Instagram Testimonies

"You have been an amazing help with info you share! I am a caregiver to the elderly and advocate for my parents and family! Thank you for everything you do, very much appreciated." -**Laura**

"I'm pretty sure that qualifies you as a real life bada$$ there Dr. Barke --- a freedom fighter and a truth teller too!" -**Dayna**

"You have so many followers because you're just that awesome!! Thanks for being there for me in my time of need. Your advice was the best! Thank you moreover for being the kind of Doctor the world needs especially at this time in our history when so many no longer trust the medical community. You are a true American Hero! Instead of a white coat you should be wearing a superhero cape. Have a great day!" -**Courtney**

"I love that I found a reputable doctor who validates my concerns about shots, toxins in our good and water! I am constantly sharing your info with anyone who will listen!! Thank you!!" -**Jenny**

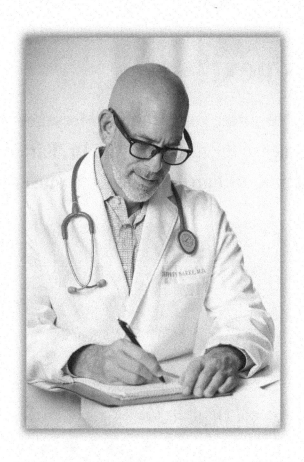

"I appreciate your honesty, and your quick response to questions. I know it must take a lot out of your day. Thank you for never making any question or concern seem silly or of no concern. I have learned so much in the last few months and I love that everyone in the community gives feedback as well. The thing I appreciate most is the encouragement to stand up for our rights, personally, legally, medically and spiritually. I work in the ER in a small hospital and it is so nice to know a doctor that thinks people have a choice about their medical health! I retire in a year and can't wait to get out. Thank you so much for all your time, effort and kindness! It is so appreciated!! God bless You!" **-Gina**

What's next?

Now that you've gotten your Morning Messages fix, take your health journey to the next level with Dr. Barke's favorite supplements, affiliated products, website and more.

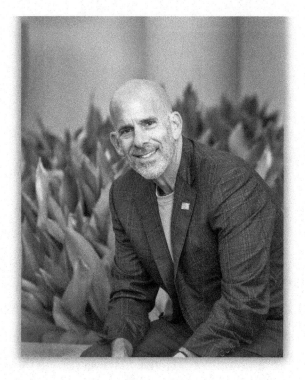

**Scan the QR & head over to
RxForLiberty.com to learn more!**

Don't forget to follow me on all socials!
@RxforLiberty

Acknowledgments:

This project was a work of love and passion but could not have been accomplished without the help and guidance of Pierce McDonnell and my son Sam Barke. Thank you to my daughter Allie Barke Quinn who pushed me to start an Instagram account several years ago and came up with the name RxForLiberty! A special thank you to my friend and critical thinker (and lay physician) Kirk Cameron for writing such a heart felt forward.

Thank you Will Witt for your friendship, wisdom, and sense of humor. Surgeon General, Joe Ladapo, your courage is inspiring - thank you for your kind words! Thank you also to holistic health coach, Stephanie Reeves, who encouraged me to question "settled" science! Finally, thank you to my social media and branding consultant Natalie Sychocka-Tucker for your guidance, inspiration, and critical eye!